Advance

MW01087926

Living
Your Joy

"These stories invite you to a place of unity and simplicity which is our natural state of being. Enjoy these amazing stories."

—Patty Luckenbach, DD,
Author of *I Only Walk On Water When It Rains*

"Since the turn of the millennium, the field of positive psychology has focused a lot on the general theme of happiness. This book highlights pure joy through diverse, well-written accounts of the writers' experiences."

—Jim Sharon, Ed.D, www.energyforlife.us
Author of *Secrets of a Soulful Marriage,*
and *Ordinary Men, Extraordinary Lives*

"A stunning collection of uplifting stories that will inspire all of us to create Joy in our lives."

—Polly Letofsky,
Author of *3mph: The Adventures of
One Woman's Walk Around the World*

"A collection of inspiring, motivating stories
of routes to joy. From letting the essence of music
imbed in our beings to the healing power of horses,
living with joy gives insight to the healing power of
living your joy."

—Anne Randolph, www.KitchenTableWriting.com
Author of an award-winning memoir,
Stories Gathered at the Kitchen Table

"Joyce has the ability to bring literature to life—hers
and others. Her previous books have moved me and
her latest venture will give all readers joy, comfort and
growth. Read slowly and savor. You will be waiting for
the next Joyce Graham offering just as I am."

—Jim Graywolf Petruzzi
Author of *White Man, Red Road, Five Colors*

"Inspiring insight in various accomplished people.
Thoughtful and warm hearted. Not fiction but true to
life experiences that anyone can relate to. Joyce Graham
hit a home run on this book and I would highly
recommend it to anyone."

—Dick Nosbisch,
Award-winning photographer
www.DickNosbisch.com

Living Your Joy

Living Your Joy

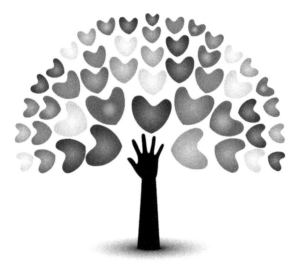

Creating a Joy-Filled Life

Edited by

Joyce Graham

Living Your Joy:
Creating a Joy-Filled Life

ISBN: 978-0-9858279-2-2
Library of Congress Control Number: 2018908570

Cover design by Nick Zelinger, NZGraphics.com
Interior design by Veronica Yager,
YellowStudiosOnline.com

"We cannot cure the world of sorrows,
but we can choose to live in joy."
—Joseph Campbell

"Joy is the holy fire that keeps our purpose
warm and our intelligence aglow."
—Helen Keller

"Sometimes your joy is the source of your smile, but
sometimes your smile can be the source of your joy."
—Nhat Hanh

Contents

Acknowledgments
i

Introduction
iii

Everyday Joy
1

The Joy of Making Music
7

On Joy
15

Calling on Joy
17

The Joy of Creation
23

Finding My BIG Joy At Burning Man
31

For the Love of Horses
39

Run to Joy
47

The Joy of Travel
53

Spiritual Joy from a Sundancers' Perspective:
An Interview with Pedro Gonzalez
59

About Joyce
65

Contributing Authors
67

Acknowledgments

For All The People who supported me during the writing of this book including the contributing authors

Judy Millyard-Maselli, Greg Nelson, Matt Michaels, Kirsten Wing, Tamara O'Dell, Sue Tanquay, Barbara Miller, David Mayes, Marion Weiss, Dr. Patty Luckenbach, Nancy Milholland.

A heart centered thank you to my contributing authors Nick Zelinger, Andrea Hall, John Candelaria, Ruth Sharon, Maura Burgess, David Karchere, Michael "Coop" Cooper, Pedro Gonzalez, Rita Roam.

Thank you for your efforts and your support. I love you all.

Introduction

Joy is what we are born for. We are called to experience the deep beauty and wonder of each day in a new way. It is the adventure of living a joy filled life that brings us happiness in all that we do. I realize that life is not always easy and strongly believe that it requires us to look at the issues we face with patience and perseverance. Finding what brings you Joy is a key to tapping into your resiliency and *your* staying power.

Mother Teresa said, "Joy is prayer; joy is strength: joy is love; joy is a net of love by which you can catch souls."

I know that what you focus on gets into your heart and mind in the most significant way. You experience and live what you think about and believe. I know this from years of Jungian training with my analyst; as well as from my mother who preached, "You become what you put into your mind so, be careful what you feed it."

So, I began meditating on the contents of this book. Could I write on Joy? Would it be inspiring and hopeful to people? Struggling with this I asked several word warriors to write about their daily experience of Joy. It really moved me how they did it. Why couldn't I do this? After being called "Joyful" by my friends for a long time where was MY Joy?

Ultimately, I did the reasonable thing. I quit my job on the military base. I left the desert of New Mexico and moved back to the pine trees and snow of Colorado.

I wrote and deleted. And, I wrote some more—most of which was challenging *until finally I found IT*. First, I awake with my morning ritual of sunrise and coffee or tea. I watch the rising sun come up, then I do Qi Gong. Next, I go for a brisk walk of at least a mile now. I have discovered that it's the adventure of starting the day that I love and *awakens* my Joy. I look forward to what will unfold and actively engage in the day to live my Joy.

This collection of Joy stories weaves together people's hearts to create a beautiful tapestry. One found her joy through her love of horses. A musician writes that his life's joy was discovered by playing in a band. Another speaks of finding joy on a walk. One experiences traveling as a gift of joy. A man finds his joy at Burning Man for the last nine years. We witness joy created in writing, a runners joy, every day joy, and finally, a poem on joy.

Every person is different, and what brings you Joy is so distinct and individual that no two people will ever experience joy in exactly the same way.

I hope you find a way to recognize your Joy as you read these essays. May you reflect on the simple truth that Joy is easily found and revealed on a daily basis. Turn within yourself, follow what you love to do, and live your joy-filled life awaiting your recognition.

Ask yourself the question "How do I create JOY in my life today?"

I wish you many Joy filled moments on your life journey.

—Joyce

Everyday Joy
by Joyce Graham

*E*very morning brings joy. Rising at 5-6 a.m., the sunrise is always unique. A new beginning to our lives. A sense of awe and wonder fills me as the blue, pink, orange colors emerge as the sun rises in the east over the trees. With a cup of tea or coffee I relax on my deck and anticipate a fresh adventure. In reverence, I welcome the joy awaiting my day.

As I write on a pad of lined paper, a little fat robin sits on the railing outside my window. It is very early spring and at this sight you know winter is slowly releasing her cold grip.

When I dive into the daily news, read the stories on social media, and listen to the troubles of the world, I have to continuously remind myself to find my comfort in simple joys. This brings a sense of peace and hope.

My Joy List

The soft Spring breeze as I take a walk outside
A loving warm embrace from my sweetheart
A thoughtfully crafted email of gratefulness
from a friend
The beauty of new buds on the trees
Colorful amusing robins on my deck
Lunch with my editor filled with good food
and laughter
The Rocky Mountains in sunlight with snow-
capped peak
A smile on the face of a stranger
Qi Gong in my living room
Cat Mandoo purring on my lap

How do I experience that we fully live more joy? By being present, aware and mindful of what brings balance to every moment. I believe being in tune with my spirit gives my life joy, authenticity and renewal each day.

One of my favorite talks by Dr. Wayne Dyer is "Inspiration." The stories he tells of living your life with purpose and heartfelt meaning are what he says can support our spirit and help us live "in spirit." Dr. Dyer also says, *"When you dance, your purpose is not to get to a certain place on the floor. It's to enjoy each step along the way."*

I love traveling. New horizons bring happiness to my life. When my parents retired, they moved to the desert southwest. I enjoyed my visits and traveling with them in their RV. I was living in Denver when I relocated for my career to this desert area and lived there for over two years. I did acclimate to the dry climate, dust storms, and the lack of trees. I realized I needed more rain, snow, and humidity to feel completely at home. I packed up and moved back to Colorado. I soon began to find my familiar place and my joy in the pine trees, ponds, and snow! We cannot live life to the fullest where the environment does not nurture our souls.

Life is not always filled with happiness. Our loved ones leave this world or leave us, our beloved pet dies, a friend moves across the country, we are let go from a job, a bad car accident changes the life of a relative, someone comes back from war a changed person. All of these things leave us in the grip of grief. None of them can be avoided. They are part of living. We have choices in how to heal and move forward. We can stay stuck. Or we can choose to find meaning and purpose again after life altering events which we achieve by connecting to that which brings us meaning and joy.

> *"One joy scatters a hundred griefs."*
> —**Chinese Proverb**

So if we embrace this Proverb, it may take only one joyful moment or experience to take away the sting of many sad ones.

Walking among the trees is what the Japanese call "Forest Bathing" or *shinrin-yoku*. It feeds who we are at the very core of our being. Forest Bathing is not about hiking or walking for exercise, but rather it is about just "being" fully present in nature. It's about taking in the sights, sounds, and smells of your surroundings with all of your senses. Breathe deeply and then exhale—just as deeply.

Shinrin-yoku allows us to totally relax and think more clearly. Connecting with nature can ease our stress and worry, restore our mood, give us back our energy and vitality, and refresh and rejuvenate us.

The thing I most enjoy about *shinrin-yoku* is that you can do it ANYwhere trees are present. In a public park, on some acreage that a friend owns, your back yard or a forest or open space. There is no agenda here. You don't have to "go" anywhere—your goal is to reconnect with your own spirit and you may even want to just lie down on the ground, do some yoga or Qi Gong, paint, or draw. Or you may just stroll around listening for the birds singing, seeing something you haven't seen before—an animal or plant, smelling the earth, feeling the bark of a tree—then bask in the awe and wonder of it all. The by-product may bring forth your unexplainable joy.

Slowing down your mind and body is essential to being present in the moment. The practice of Mindfulness brings us into the awareness of our thoughts, feelings, bodily sensations, and surrounding environment while practicing a state of non-judgment. Mindfulness means being fully in the "present" rather than projecting into the future or remaining attached to the past. We pay attention to our thoughts, but we do not judge them. There is no "right" or "wrong" way to think or feel in any given moment.

My hope is that we are asking ourselves in our daily lives how to serve our community, how to help a beloved friend, our spouse may need something, a neighbor has a problem with grief. We stretch ourselves a little and ask how we may help bridge this need with grace and joy.

Joy is what we are here to explore and experience as we walk this life path in our own unique ways.

Joseph Campbell was popular when I was in graduate school and we discussed his theory based on his belief that we must "follow our bliss." We must look for the signs and concur within ourselves that which is our life-calling. It takes work to be consciously aware of our lives moment to moment. But isn't that the blessing—to recognize it, to know it, and live it?

What will bring your heart joy and how can you live it? "Heart math" has evidence that our heart energy to expands to up to 50 feet around our bodies. The more love and joy we carry in our hearts the more we expand this and share this energy with others.

Won't you join me in the journey to start noticing even the smallest things in your world that will bring you joy and subsequently expand your heart energy with those you encounter?

Sources

[1] Wayne Dyer: You Tube Video "Motivation"
[2] Forest Bathing, article from Time Magazine:
   http://time.com/5259602/japanese-forest-bathing/

About Joyce

Joyce Graham, MS, LPC is an author, presenter, Licensed Professional Counselor, and Qi Gong Instructor with over thirty years of experience. Her previous books include The Healer, a novel and The Path: Herbs, Homeopathy, Holistic Healing.

Visit her at www.JoyceGraham.com or on her YouTube Channel.

The Joy of Making Music
by Nick Zelinger

"The reason I play music is to touch people—for selfish reasons, as well.

It feels good to make someone else feel something, whether it's a kiss, a painting, a good idea or a song."
— **Dave Matthews**[1]

W hen I first started singing in bands as a teenager, there were multiple reasons why I did so: I wanted to be part of a group (something larger than myself); I wanted to be popular and liked; I wanted to express myself with my voice; and probably a host of other reasons, big and small.

But before I seriously decided to make music a career, I had been singing (along to records, in church choirs, and on street corners with like-minded vocalists) for the pure joy of it. At the time, I never gave much thought to any deep reason or intent—it simply felt wonderful and uplifting.

I was blessed to have a family that loved to sing. Both my mother and father had wonderful singing voices. At an early age, I could recognize the joy they had in singing along to the radio or a song on the record player. While they weren't technically proficient, they exuded warmth, excitement, their joy—each time they lifted their voices in song.

I suspect it's not much different with anyone who makes music—at any level. Singing or playing an instrument tends to raise endorphins, accelerate our heart rate—and open up our hearts to the many emotions we convey in song.

> *"Music is a moral law. It gives soul to the universe, wings to the mind, flight to the imagination, and charm and gaiety to life and to everything."*
>
> —Plato[1]

At an early age, I realized I could hold a tune, and found singing a wonderful expression of generating emotions of all kinds. Now in my sixties—and still performing—I have a better appreciation for the modest skills I have developed. I learned to play guitar and piano on my own. Granted, those skills are very limited compared to the dedicated musicians who have labored to perfect their art. But, learning to play instruments gave me the ability to eventually compose my own music and perform for audiences. I've known no greater joy (next to becoming a parent) than to express my art and know, in some instances, that I've affected someone's heart with my music.

As for me, hearing a choir or vocal ensemble sing is still the most thrilling, uplifting experience. I love and appreciate all genres of music, and hearing a choral work like "O magnum mysterium" composed by Morten Lauridsen, never ceases to astound me with the knowledge that the human voice raised in song can produce such spiritual magnificence. Next to nature—the song of birds—nothing seems as monumental.

The joy of performing music comes, in part, from the preparation: the hours, weeks, and years of practice, and endless rehearsals. In this way, it is no different than any sport. They both require training, making mistakes, learning new skills and repetition. And of course, performance.

When I was in college, the rock band I was in was popular enough to be asked on several occasions to open for national acts. On one such night, we opened for the iconic 60's band, Vanilla Fudge. They had a megahit with "You Keep Me Hanging On." We performed A 30-40 minute set before a crowd of 10,000 people.

Nervous but excited, we were young enough not to feel intimidated. We also had a lot of confidence, having started the band in high school and continuing on into college. I have a crystal clear moment of performing a couple of songs that were greeted with great enthusiasm: covers of the Doors' "The Crystal Ship" and Procol Harum's "Whiter Shade of Pale."

The exuberance I felt not only of performing for such a large, loud crowd, but also of knowing I was singing and playing well has stayed with me to this day. There have been many other such times through the years, where the song, the performance, the crowd, all coalesced in making such moments magical and even transcending.

Music can indeed transform the performer and the listener—they both become part of a special community where both share in the creation and the appreciation of a performance. I've known performing music to lift me from a deep depression to the highest of joyful peaks— all within the space of a 3-minute song.

"Your personal history is a part of what happens with your hands and your head as you play music."
—**Dave Grohl**[1]

On many occasions—too countless to mention, the pure magic of playing music with other musicians resulted in being transported to another realm. Like athletes, it is referred to as being "in the zone", where everyone in the band is clicking on all cylinders: The drummer and bass player are locked into the solid beat; the keyboard, rhythm guitar player and lead guitarist are all playing at their peak. Everyone is listening to and playing off each other. It is a creative, symbiotic relationship that reaps mounds of benefits and enjoyment.

Likewise, in the recording studio; the joy of creating one's own music is an enticing, almost addictive experience. Having been a songwriter for years, I've continually honed my craft. When the opportunity came to record the first album with the band, Saxxon Woods— a 6 piece band—all of whom were singer songwriters— the excitement and anticipation were almost beyond control.

Collaborating with the other band members and recording engineer was one of the most exciting times in my life. Not only was everyone a gifted and skilled musician and vocalist, but our common goal was to create a collection of well-crafted songs that we had created and rehearsed for months. When it came time to record the initial tracks, we had already created arrangements for vocals and instruments that we were convinced were sound and sturdy.

"Music is intangible and ephemeral, but it comes from the home world of the spirit, and though so fleeting, it is recognized by the spirit as a soul-speech fresh from the celestial realms,

*an echo from the home whence we are now
exiled, and therefore it touches a cord in our
being, regardless of whether we realize the true
cause or not."*

—Max Heindel[2]

So it should come as no surprise to anyone who has performed music, whether it be Classical, Folk, Rock, Jazz, Rap; or any of the myriad of styles and genres across the globe—that it is a uplifting soul-searching, and spiritual experience.

And that goes for ANYONE making music—at any skill level, it can be enjoyed, shared, nurtured and used for self-healing and the common good.

In the words of Sean Combs, "Music is the most powerful form of communication in the world. It brings us all together. Even religion separates us, but a hit record unites us across religious beliefs, race, and politics."[2]

Sources

[1] http://www.brainyquote.com/quotes/keywords/
play_music.html

[2] http://www.brainyquote.com/quotes/topics/topic_
music7.html

About Nick

Nick Zelinger spent 20 years as a touring musician, taught himself guitar, keyboards and bass guitar; opening for such music legends as The Vanilla Fudge, Strawberry Alarm Clock, and J.J. Cale. He recorded 3 albums with the eclectic folk rock band, Saxxon Woods. He continues to revel in the joys of making music, performing with the Denver-based rock band, Thin Ice (www.ThinIceBand.com).

Nick's has a successful career as a book designer, winning numerous national and international book awards (www.NZGraphics.com).

Nick is also the co-author, along with Tammy Brackett, of the award-winning book Another Nightmare Gig from Hell, true stories from musicians across the country. *It is available on Amazon in softcover, eBook, and now in AudioBook format.*

On Joy
by John J. Candelaria

Joy lives inside us and often will fill
moments in time, a delight in being
alive to see a Morning Glory spill
unrestricted beauty ever stunning.

We accept the joy of caring for others,
fully engage in this practice, happy
to give all without reward or favors,
a style of living with great jubilee.

When distress enters our order in life,
a sad time prevails seemly forever.
Those seasons of turmoil and strife
give way as the sounds of joy gain tenure.

Host delight first in yourself, then take pride
in times joy turns into a great joyride.

About John

John J. Candelaria describes himself as a narrative poet who enjoys writing poetry to capture the sound of language. In postic lines and free verse his poems have been published in The Storyteller's Anthology, *Southwest Writers,* The Oasis Journal 2012 *and* 2013, *in the anthology,* Poetry From The Other Side: an anthology, *Albuquerque chapter, New Mexico State Poetry Society, and in the Southwest Sage newsletter of the SouthWest Writers.*

Calling on Joy
by Ruth Sharon

*O*ne summer morning, I was strolling along a lovely nature path, feeling very grateful and relaxed. My breathing was slow and rhythmic and my body felt light. The subtle grip of tension in my belly was gone. What a freedom to be present in the moment!

I named this freeing feeling *Joy*, as if this quality is a person. She appeared in my imagination as radiant, energetic, delighted, kind and warm. I saw her dressed in a golden sundress, with light shimmering on her hair, eyes wide open and glistening, and a smile that exudes from her inner glow. I felt her walk beside me, on this nature path, through the expanse of shade trees and winding stream. What an abundant and grateful way to live, with Joy at the side! I rededicated myself right then and there to align with heart-opening Joy as often as I can remember.

In that moment, I realized that Joy is available at all times. I can just call on her. **JOY is juicy, open, youthful.** I pledge to myself to not allow joy to be covered over and inaccessible, even during distressing times. After all, the sun is still shining, even on a cloudy day.

I acknowledge that joy is much more than a feeling; it is a state of being, a view of the world, a way of life. *Joy* has her own vibration, an energy frequency. She is the womb I grow within, a luminous vessel for my life. She can be the very air I breathe, the atmosphere that surrounds and permeates me, just as Love does.

When I am most conscious, I adore the realization that the true essence in my heart is inner peace and joy. Even in dark times, during difficult situations, I can call on *Joy* as the illuminator to reflect the inner light and reveal the deeper purpose of the situation. She can give meaning to my discomfort, so as to quicken my learning the given lesson or unveiling the hidden message. What a friend *Joy* is!

As I recognize my growth/dormancy cycles and layers of conditioned fears, Joy is with me. I thank her for encouraging me to open to and trust the Divine Dance. To me, she is the embodiment of the Divine Feminine. I dance with her as I journey through life.

I am so humbled to live in this time when genuine joy is more acceptable and openly celebrated. With rapidly-evolving consciousness, I, along with many others, am moving from survival to activating true soul purpose.

My husband of 45 years, Jim Sharon, and I are on this soul's journey together. I have joked with him that I spent my childhood preparing for him, and when I met him in college at 19, I knew him! What a marvel to be able to connect on all levels of our being. Regularly, I feel as if I am still a young maiden, dating my boyfriend! Doing the most mundane household chores can be fun and sexy. Cleaning our closets and flirting, as we honor the change of seasons, we acknowledge as a "date." Having dates in our house and out in the world are ways we love to be together without distractions. Praying and meditating each morning and evening is a lovely way we *bookend* our days together.

Delighting in my three grown children, their partners and two grandchildren (so far), I am continually amazed how we all keep growing individually and as a family.

Recently, dear friends visited, one of whom I had not seen for over 30 years!

To pick up right where we left off is such a warm feeling in my heart and soul. We shared a conversation about how our soul purpose is being revealed to us on a daily basis. Such a rich moment—I expand my usual reality into the cosmos and then back into my body! As a spiritual being having a human experience, I am in humble acceptance of the magic of this creation!

Spending time in nature always gives me the space to just *be*. I may simply be having a cup of tea or a meal in my backyard, listening to the birds and crickets. I may ride into the mountains for a hike or a few days' retreat. Exploring the elements of earth, air, fire and water allows Joy to be at my side. Meditating by the ocean or a stream brings me a sense of peace and contentment as I experience unity with the All. Soaking in hot mineral baths is one of my favorite ways to enter the sacred waters of the Mother Earth. Receiving delight through my senses is so renewing for my spirit and connection. My mind is quiet, there is only the present moment. I exhale deeply and know I am safe, enveloped in love and forever blessed.

At those times, *Joy* is very apparent; at other times, she is beyond my conscious awareness. Dealing with difficult moments can be so challenging. Being reactive and stressed diminishes my ability to be present and clear. Breathing slowly and deeply, I calm myself and allow the healing power of the Divine to suffuse me. This spiritual practice of bringing love to pain is a sweet, sublime joy. It is the knowing that I am facing what is in my life at the moment with as much love as I can.

I recently returned from an out of town visit with my 94-year old mother. Being with my dear mom is so bittersweet. Reminiscing about my childhood is fun, yet her short-term memory is so vacant. I had to remind myself to bring alive joy in the tiny moments. Being in a new nursing home is scary and uncomfortable for her, much like my first days in the college dorm. I encourage her to enjoy her meals and activities, all the while, addressing some of her real concerns about the end of her life. Facing the reality of her diminishing functioning and returning to child-like dependency is so sad. Holding the joy and the sadness in my heart has been painful and is leading to deep healing about her mortality, and my own.

When I was a young child I remember sitting on the doorstep of our new house, in deep concentration. My mother came outside and asked me what I was doing. I said "I am loving all the people in the houses on my street. I love everyone, even people I don't know." She smiled, patted my head, and later recounted the story to my father when he came home from work.

My life purpose is to bring more love and joy into this world! I am a Warrior for Love! I aspire to create safe space to let down defenses and open more rooms in the Mansion of Love! Marriage has been a living laboratory for me to discover my true nature and clear off the layers of limiting beliefs and fears. I keep learning how committed love brings true freedom to be myself. Joy encompasses all my other feelings. I can feel the joy of telling the truth about what I am feeling, where I hurt, how I long to be.

Leaving a legacy to the next generations is essential to me. I pray that I am a model of living a conscious, mindful, joyful life. Our daughter is married to a terrific guy and has two lovely daughters. Watching my younger granddaughter start pre-school is such a delight. She is reveling in all the new toys, people and activities. She keeps shrieking, "Fun! fun! fun!" My older granddaughter and I are very close. We share a love of yoga, among other interests. Several years ago, we collaborated on a three-generation yoga book, along with my younger daughter.

Expressing myself in words, storytelling, songs, dancing, yoga, cooking, art and serving others satisfies a deep need in me to generously share wisdom and soul. I call on Joy and she comes, blessing me with peace. I am grateful for my life!

About Ruth

Ruth Sharon, M.S. is a Licensed Professional Counselor, Registered Yoga Teacher and Sufi Healing Conductor. She and her husband Dr. Jim Sharon live in Centennial, CO and enjoy being with their family, friends and community.

Ruth and Jim have joyfully collaborated in writing the book Secrets of a Soulful Marriage: Creating and Sustaining A Loving, Sacred Relationship, *SkyLight Paths Publishing, 2014. They offer personal counseling, as well as Coaching for Soulful Couples and Singles, retreats, seminars and a myriad of articles and interviews. They are voted "Best Relationship Coaches" in 2015 and 2016.*

Visit Ruth at: www.energyforlife.us

The Joy of Creation
by David Karchere

For me, the joy of creation comes in so many forms. Creating a family with my wife, Joyce, and raising our daughter, Helena, was one of the most fulfilling experiences of my life. Creating a barbecue picnic for friends is incredible fun. (Irma Rombauer didn't call her cookbook The Joy of Cooking for nothing!) And there are other experiences, too numerous to count.

One of the most ecstatic experiences of creation I have had is in songwriting. When I first began, it was with guitar in hand, working out the words, the melody and the chords. Later I wrote the notes with a pencil on staff paper. For the past twenty years, I've been writing the music on a computer program that lets me drop the notes on the staff with a mouse and then play them through a synthesizer.

However, I've done it, the experience has been the same. There is the physical part of it—the pencil, the paper, and later the computer and the mouse—but that's not where the major part of the creation is occurring. I go on an inner journey that is truly the act of creation.

I enter a dark room in consciousness. I am listening, more and more deeply. I am feeling the very air of that dark place. Soon there are waves of feeling and meaning, with a rhythm all to themselves, that form in the air. They grow in strength and intensity, one after another, landing in my heart and mind. They are saying something so profoundly beautiful, yet heartbreaking and excruciatingly poignant, crashing over me one after another. I ask the waves to say what they have to say again so that I can record it on paper or on my computer screen.

> *Long ago, far away,*
> *Bathed in gold,*
> *Was a place that shown in sunlit glow.*
> *I remember that regal splendor,*
> *How warm and tender,*
> *My love and I..*
> *Those peaceful hours,*
> *The quiet rivers,*
> *Among wild flowers,*
> *My love and I.*

(From my song, *I Remember*.)

There is a craft to writing songs. There is a working of harmonic patterns, melodies and rhymes. But far more important is the opportunity to enter that dark place and know the rhythms of creation and all their meaning.

The true nature of joy so often eludes us. So how we experience joy is a vital topic for anyone. I believe it deserves a deeply philosophical examination as well as a heightened intuitive awareness.

Witnessing others and observing the world at large, it is easy to see people looking for joy in all the wrong places. Drugs and alcohol are perhaps the most obvious examples of dead ends in the search for joy—but not the only ones. Advertising has become a modern-day oracle in a futile search for joy. It entices people to extract joy out of virtually every facet of human experience— everything from cars to sex to Coca-Cola—until there is no more joy left to extract.

I don't want to spend too much time railing against our culture. But I think it helps to appreciate how constantly anyone who is plugged into the mass media is assailed by these false messages. So many of them are a promise of joy "if only..."

Then there is our own personal experience. I've learned that I can be joy-averse—that I can default to a way of living that endures the more difficult experiences that come to me and looks for some relief from that, but doesn't make room for real pleasure and deep joy.

Living, by its very nature, has its up and downs. We are all riding the great sine wave of life. In the natural world, the tide ebbs and flows. There is the great cycle of life in which mineral substance is lifted up to form plants and animals, and then returned to the earth. That cycle includes both birth and death.

In our own experience, we sometimes have a kind of tragic human drama that we bring to the natural cycles of life. Sometimes we human beings imprint our own craziness on them. So much so, that it is hard to imagine what would be truly natural for us without the insanity of all the plagues that humanity has brought to the world—terrorism and war, nuclear bombs and global warming and more. And then, at a personal level, resentment and retribution, envy and depression.

The path to joy can seem to be all about riding the upward-moving oscillation of the sine wave. More happiness. More enlightenment. More pleasure. Less pain.

There are so many personal agendas that promise to take us there. Everything from personal development workshops to a trip to the Bahamas to earning more money to becoming more spiritual. Think positive! Ride the upward part of the sine wave to the top! Just like the Cyclone roller coaster at Coney Island! What a view!

The incoming tide in the cycles of life is exhilarating. It buoys us up and brings a thrill. I am all for more happiness, more enlightenment, more pleasure and less pain. And I've always wanted to vacation in the Bahamas. But there is a great distinction between the happiness to be experienced surfing on the incoming tide and the deeper reality of joy. And what goes up must come down.

Real joy is not the happiness a person tries to extract from life. It isn't a temporary high. Real joy is the joy of creation. *Creation* is a marvelous word. It is a thing—a specific thing that you or I create. It can also be *everything*—the whole world. The universe!

Creation is also an act. And again, it can be any act of creation, from painting a picture to the act of creating everything.

Where there is creation, there is a creator. That could be you or me, or both of us together. It could be all of us together—*all humanity*. It can also be *the* Creator; the God, by whatever name, that is at the heart of the atom, at the heart of a human being, and within all of Creation.

At every level, there is the joy of creation. The joy of the substance of creation—including our own physical bodies. The joy of being animated by the power of creation in the incredible design of creation. And joy in the process of creation.

That process includes flood tides and ebb tides. It includes the substance of creation coming together and rising up, and it includes the decay of that substance so that it descends to a lower level.

Here is a fun philosophical question that has a surprising, yet profound answer. Imagine that you were the great God of the Universe. You don't even have to believe in God to try this out. Imagine yourself in the deep black of space with no creation. Just you. And then you have this brilliant idea:

I could create a universe! I could create nebulae, stars and planets. I could use my amazing creative power to manifest something magnificent! I could create planet Earth with conditions that promote life-forms of all kinds. I could even create a life-form that could become conscious of me who is doing all this.

Here is the philosophical question: If you were the great God of the Universe, thinking those thoughts, what would be your motivation for creating the universe and everything in it? For creating planet Earth and everything upon it, including human beings?

I have found only one answer that makes any sense to me. Only for the joy of creation.

In that empty space before creation, there was no problem to solve. There was nothing to improve. If there was any reason at all for creating, the only one I can imagine is joy.

I propose that this is also the only reason for a human life. Yes, there are many expressions of that one reason. Yes, we surf all the ups and downs of the sine wave of life; the pleasure and some pain.

In a song made famous by Garth Brooks, songwriter, Tony Arata says it this way:

Our lives are better left to chance,
I could have missed the pain,
But I'd have had to miss the dance.

The reason for a human life is not just about the ups or the downs, the pleasure and the pain. It is about the glory of it all.

The joy of creation is tuning into something that is, at first, only essence—an unmanifest potential—and letting it take form. It is so magical when it does. The magic is different depending on the nature of the essence and the form that embodies it. The root of the joy is the same.

Your joy may be watching your baby smiling up at you while she lies in her crib. Or listening to your own original song whose passionate melody expresses that mad love in your own heart. It could be the smile on the face of a friend as they eat a spare rib that you marinated and baked and grilled.

The root of the word *joy* is the Latin word *gaudere*. It means rejoice. So rejoice in all creation—even the downs, as well as the ups. Real joy is rejoicing in it all, just like I imagine the great God of the Universe must have done on that first day of creation long ago, and even today.

You are a creator. When you know that deeply for yourself, and you live it every day in even the most mundane of moments, no one can take it away from you.

No matter what happens, you have the joy of that knowing.

About David

David Karchere is an author, speaker, poet, workshop leader and foremost thought leader on Primal Spirituality worldwide. David has created and led unique workshops for spiritual awakening and personal transformation for people around the globe. He has also developed The Creative Field Project, a global network of small groups that meet to further the work of Primal Spirituality. David has just finished writing his first book, Becoming a Sun: Emotional and Spiritual Intelligence for a Happy, Fulfilling Life.

David is a member of the Evolutionary Leaders group. His home is Sunrise Ranch in Loveland, Colorado, U.S.A., a teaching and demonstration site for Primal Spirituality.

Visit David at: www.davidkarchere.com

Finding My BIG Joy At Burning Man
by Michael "Coop" Cooper

*M*any people search for joy in small ways in their everyday lives, which I whole heartedly encourage. I personally access my joy in a completely *BIG* way for two weeks every year. Don't get me wrong, I experience joy in my daily life, but my *BIG* Joy comes from a crazy festival that takes place once a year in the desert of Nevada called Burning Man!

Every year, for the past nine years, Burning Man is my pilgrimage, my refuge, my vacation and my vocation. I find my joy because it pours out of me here. I keep going back because it renews me.

No matter what you've heard about this festival, it pales in comparison to actually attending the Real Deal. For two weeks, I volunteer to lead a diverse crew of artists, craftsmen, carpenters, builders, plumbers, electricians and a slew of other volunteers and we build a part of the temporary city of 68,000 people that we lovingly refer to as Black Rock City. It's built on a vast, flat, open desert plain and when we arrive, there is literally nothing there—for miles!

It's an extreme environment with dust storms, wind, scorching heat and unpredictable weather—this year it even got below freezing at night in August! So, why does this crazed environment bring me joy?

First, it's a complete departure from my normal day-to-day reality. My schedule is up to me—no one else dictates what I have to do or where I have to be. I'm totally free to explore my creativity. As the volunteer leader for a 150-person camp, I'm in charge of everything, which is exhilarating and fun because I get to solve problems and puzzles all day long—*and* I get the final say!

Burning Man is a festival of *living art*; everyone wears costumes, so it's rare to find someone in normal clothes. We use our imaginativeness to transform ourselves into works of art and express our creativity through our costumes. It's a feast for the eyes—one that brings a wide smile to my face almost all day every day. To see people of all ages and shapes and sizes exploring aspects of themselves that have likely remained dormant since childhood is a magical experience. Just a bunch of folks being kids again creates a Wonderland in this desert oasis.

After we build our camp—complete with hot showers, a commercial kitchen that serves 300 hot meals a day, a 1200 square foot dining lounge for our campers and venues for entertainment, including an aerial rig, a stage with spotlights and sound, a full-service gym, a small gathering spot for musicians to play and a giant orange dome with 50-foot-tall stalks from the top that we call the Carrot Dome filled with nets for lounging— we surround our entire camp with colorful day-glow flags and fill our courtyard with large-scale kinetic art sculptures. It's a beautiful, 24-hour playground filled with love and inspiration.

I find my joy here. I've been going for so many years, that dozens of friends stop by each day to catch up, marvel at our art installations, join us for gourmet meals, take in a show from our performers and even help us clean up our dishes. It's community-fueled love and friendship at its best.

After our camp is set up, I get to explore the art, the music, the food, the ingenuity and the beauty of this desert plain full of eager participants who are always having fun! It really is like being a kid again, totally free, following wherever our hearts desire, interacting with total strangers with warm embraces and hearty laughter. It can be bawdy and serene and festive and quiet. I embrace all these things to fully experience Burning Man.

The desert floor is called "the playa". At night it fills with lights and art cars and whacky revelers who are on their mad adventures until sun up. The colors, the lights, the sounds, the vast open spaces with thousands of people are a cacophony of craziness that renews my spirit, inspires me to create, renews my faith in humanity and warms my soul.

While the extreme conditions can keep many people away, it's a welcoming enclave for the adventurous, the free, the seekers, the artists, the explorers, and the lovers in us all. I've never experienced the type of warmth and comfort anywhere else and I've traveled the world.

My first year, I arrived in the middle of the night, eager and wide-eyed, only knowing one other person in our camp. I was a bit nervous, but excited! I set up my tent and started talking to other members, who quickly offered me help and a cocktail. It was 6 am when the sun was just coming up. I didn't know what to expect, but I was determined to stay present and take it all in. I was surrounded by art and costumes, trying to get my bearings—all the while a goofy wide smile was plastered on my face.

I finished setting up my tent and started getting my bike ready for an adventure. Within a few minutes, I heard a loud noise—it was a siren coming from a megaphone about 20 feet away. At first, I was startled, thinking it was an emergency vehicle, but to my surprise, it was a signal from our camp organizer. Every morning at 7am, they all got together for a dance break to kick off the day! It took me a few minutes to warm up, but I could feel the kid spirit in me start to emerge. This fun free-style aerobics led into a most glorious day, where I got to know new people and explored the playa with a new group of fantastic friends.

Around noon that day, a huge dust storm swept across the playa. We had arrived back in camp after checking out several art installations—just in time for my first white out. I literally couldn't see my hand in front of my face. The wind howled, the dust blew and I thought we would be "stuck," immobile for hours. One of our campmates, wearing googles and a dust mask found our stereo system and turned it up full blast. What could have been a really scary and dangerous experience ANYwhere else, magically turned into a dance party on the playa! Within a few minutes, there were 20 people dancing on our dance floor, swirling and swaying in the dust. For about two hours, people came in and out, literally appearing on the floor and disappearing a few minutes later, laughing, dancing and having a great time. I've never had as many hugs as I did during that dust storm. Complete strangers heard the music and were attracted like moths to a flame. Every single one of them thanked us for the music and wished us, "A great burn"

A few days later, after way too much fun, I got separated from my campmates and got a little confused about where I was. I started to panic—It almost felt like when I was lost in the grocery store at four-years-old. My heart started racing. I looked around to try to get my bearings, but nothing looked familiar. I was a little sleep-deprived, a little dehydrated and exhausted. I didn't know what to do. Thankfully I had my bike, so I decided to ride around a bit and figure out where I was and look for my new friends. I couldn't find them anywhere, but right by the side of the road was this terrific looking red sofa. As I rolled up to it, three smiling faces asked me to sit with them. One was from Amsterdam, one was from France and the other was from Australia. None of them knew each other, but were attracted to the fantastic red sofa. They offered me water and a big hug. After a few minutes, they asked if I was up for an adventure. A smile crept across my face. I said, "Sure!" I totally forgot that I was already a little lost.

We jumped on our bikes and headed toward the sound of some great music. Within a few minutes, we were on a dance floor, smiling, laughing and getting to know each other. As I was dancing, I turned around and bumped into my other friends that I had lost earlier! They screeched, gave me hugs and said they missed me. On the playa, we have a saying, "The playa provides."

While this is only one small illustration of how "the playa provides," it has happened again and again.

I have one last story for you. A couple of years ago, I was in charge of our camp water, gray water and infrastructure. One night, in the dark, someone accidentally poured some graywater into our fresh water tank. That contaminated all 1,000 gallons of fresh water that we had. This was an emergency situation—150 people were without fresh water. A campmate woke me up at 7am to explain the situation and I bolted out of bed, knowing that we only had a few hours to avert a crisis situation.

I had to find water and fast. I jumped on my bike in search of our water supplier. Normally, whenever biking on the playa, it's important to carry water to drink, but because all of our water was contaminated, I had to go without. I ventured a block or two and stopped, having no idea where to go or how to find them. Sweat started to pour off my brow. I had an awful sinking feeling in the pit of my stomach. I started to panic. Once again, I felt like a four-year-old, completely lost and utterly frightened. So, I decided to ask for help. I looked up at the sky and said, "Please guide me to the water truck." I indisputably heard, "Take a right," so I turned my bike right and pedaled for a few blocks. Once again I stopped and asked, "Where to now?" That time I heard, "In two blocks, take a left." So, I biked up two blocks and as I turned left, the water truck was also turning onto the street right in front of me. I started to shake, feeling overwhelmingly elated. I was giddy with excitement as I glided up beside the truck and waived the driver down to ask him for help. He radioed his dispatcher and had a truck out to replace our contaminated tank, pump and filter within two hours— before most of our camp was awake and was even aware that we had a water problem. Crisis averted. This type of magical experience happens all the time on playa.

"The playa provides." Indeed!

I hope one day, you'll join me on the playa and that we have a serendipitous encounter so that I get to see the joy pour out of your eyes and your smile as it does mine. This place is delightfully *enchanted*. Will you allow yourself to find your joy here?

About Michael

Michael O. "Coop" Cooper is an internationally recognized executive coach, advisor, facilitator and trainer from San Francisco, California. He specializes in helping right-brain entrepreneurs recognize and monetize their brilliance to grow their companies. He founded Innovators + Influencers to help business leaders learn the skills, tools and strategies to thrive in a constantly changing environment. Even though he loves his work, he sneaks away for two weeks to the Burning Man festival in the Nevada Black Rock Desert every year to renew his spirit.

Visit Michael at: www.innovatorsandinfluencers.com

For the Love of Horses
by Andrea M. Hall

I was raised as a city girl, if you consider a town of 30,000 a city! Yet I always had a passion for horses. As a child, I would go to visit my mother's side of the family, who were farmers and we would get to ride horses. I didn't get to do it very often, yet when I did it was pure pleasure. Being a child riding horses is much different than being an adult riding horse. You get on without a care in the world and don't pay much attention to the potential danger of this 1500-pound animal. You are very resilient as a child and can bounce back very easy. As an adult, not so much!

In my late 20's, I decided I was going to go for a ride one day on a friend's horse, as I really wanted to be around these beautiful creatures again. I had recently broken up with my boyfriend and I was not in a good space. I was bound and determined to go for a ride.

Little did I know, this horse was going to take me for a ride of his own. I have since learned and discovered how horses feed off of our energy and mine was not good. While sitting on the back of the horse my root chakra was directly connected to their will and determination chakra and when those two are not in alignment it can only mean one thing TROUBLE!

While saddling up the horse I could tell he wasn't listening and was pulling away from me. I had no clue— I just thought the horse was being "naughty". While out for a stroll the horse was not listening to me again and just STOPPED. In my eagerness to ride, I was determined to get him to listen to me. I began to kick him to get him to continue along the fence line and instead he whipped around and took off. In order to stay on the back of the horse I squeezed my thighs to try and hold on. In the horse world that means go faster and faster he went. Eventually I could hold on no longer and I ended up getting dumped in the middle of the pasture. While lying there thinking how did this happen, the horse came back at me and I thought for sure that I was about to die. By the grace of God this horse either went around me or over me. Not sure as my eyes were closed and I was praying for help. As I lay in the pasture and wonder how was I ever going to get back to the barn the horse made his way back to the barn without me.

Helped arrived shortly and after a long visit at the emergency room I found myself in a wheel chair with a broken pelvis and shattered arm. After numerous surgeries and 6 months in a wheel chair I once again found myself craving the warmth of this 4-legged animal again.

My mother thought I was crazy, as would most people. My mom continued to encourage me to find another passion one that was "less dangerous" in her words. She was scared that I would once again get hurt yet I knew better. There was something down deep that was once again calling me to be close to these animals. Don't get me wrong it took me several years to get the confidence to get back on a horse and be in their presence without fear. However, over time and facing my fears I was able to accomplish this.

I moved to Colorado and decided it was time to feel their unconditional love again. I began riding and taking time to just "BE" in their presence. I started doing some personal growth work that involved horses and discovered how connected I was with myself when I was around them. I felt my world melt and disappear. Hours would pass and it felt like minutes until I left the barn and discovered time had not stood still. My breathing pattern would change, I would become less anxious and more relaxed. I was grounded, peaceful and felt right at home. The minute I would leave and go back to the real world I would crave that feeling and wanted to bottle it up for when I was at home away from the barn.

I knew that I had found my place. Yet like most people I went back to the world I knew the constant drive and determination of worldly things and my job. Well for me, my job was literally killing me. I had become ill and was doing anything and everything to figure it out. I did as many natural and holistic things as I could. If you had told me to stand on my head and you will feel better I would have done it.

After three years of searching for an answer I caved and went to see a western medicine doctor. The funny thing about that is, at first glance he too told me there was nothing the matter with me as I had passed all the neurological tests. He said we can do an MRI yet I don't think it will show anything. So, I left and another 6 weeks went by before I said no I will do the MRI. I had to have some answers. Then began the insurance fight as they believed I still had not done enough to warrant a MRI to be covered by insurance.

After jumping through all their circus hoops I was allowed the MRI. Within 20 minutes of completing the MRI my life would forever be changed. I received the dreaded news…I had a brain tumor. My world went silent. Did I just hear that correctly? A brain tumor. People who have those die, right? I am pretty sure I didn't hear much after that.

My everyday life turned into a 4-alarm fire. As a lawyer I went into task mode and started putting my life together on sheets of paper. I didn't know if after surgery I would wake up and hear I am okay or you have "cancer". My life was literally in limb bow. I vowed that day that if I was given a second chance at life that I would take it and do something different. I would choose to live my life so differently.

After surgery, I received a Christmas Miracle. It wasn't cancer and I would be just fine. After several longs months of recovery and laying in my bed thinking 'what will I do differently?' I once again went back to what brought me such joy and it was my love for horses and how they can help heal. I began to do as much as I could with the horses and be around then as much as possible. I figured out how to heal and let go of so many things that were holding me back in my life. It helped me discover me again!

I just recently got married and after running around planning the wedding for the past 6 months I forgot how to be in my body and get out of my head. I went back to where I knew I could be grounded and centered, with my horses. I walked out to the pasture and for the first time in a long time I could once again feel my body just melt. I felt my heart beat, my shoulders relaxed and got back into my body. I went 'WOW' this is what that feels like. I just stood in the presence of "Bugs" our horse that stand 17 plus hands high. That's horse talk for almost 6 feet tall. He might be big yet he has the biggest heart one could imagine. He just stood next to me heart to heart and filled my depleted energy tank. It brought me to tears and then laughter before we parted ways for the afternoon.

These creatures give to this world unconditionally every day. They have traveled this world and been used for work, war and pleasure and ask for nothing in return other than love. Truth be told. They give us more love than we could ever give them. No strings attached as they live in the present moment unlike us human beings. The horse doesn't live with regret or remember that you were 10 minutes late to feed the day before. They are right here in the here and now. They keep me in that space if even just for a moment in time. If I forget they will quickly remind me by stepping on a toe to say 'hey, check back in'.

If you have never experienced the love of a horse or the joy it can bring just by being in their presence, I ask that you find a horse rescue or anyone with horses and just observe their behavior. See how you feel and what happens in your own body while standing in their presence. I can tell you they are not just my horse they are my therapist, stability, joy and most importantly my BEST FRIEND! "Let the whisper of the horse echo the spirit of the soul." ®

About Andrea

Andrea M. Hall is a certified Equine Gestalt Coach. She earned her certification through Melisa Pearce's program "Touched By A Horse". Through her own healing she and her horses are working with lawyers who may be at a crossroads in their life or just wanting to get off the hamster wheel of life. Couples who are struggling and wanting to determine what the next step in their relationship looks like. People who just want to heal old wounds and want to bring more peace and balance into their lives.

She has owned and operated a successful law firm specializing in sex offenses and domestic violence. Andrea is also a speaker and author of *Sex and Justice*. "*Let the whisper of the horse echo the spirit of the soul.*"®

Visit Andrea at: www.witherswhisper.com

Run to Joy
by Rita Roem

*F*or a brief and glorious two years, I was a runner. I ran for forty to fifty minutes a day, 6 or 7 days a week. I was not a gym runner. I ran outside, and didn't let the weather stop me. Modern technology has made that easy. It took me time to work up to 50 minutes. 20 was all I could do at first, but I added at least one minute to my time each time I ran. My colleagues/friends were runners, and they helped me get started: my cheerleaders. I had a job at that time that was, in comparison to my previous job, stress-free. I had time on my hands. The Internet was still too young to consume much time, and I lived in a place of beauty. I was single and 36.

I lived on the campus of an international high school in Eastern Europe. It was built in the 1860's on park-like grounds where each season produced its own form of beauty. It was a great place to be a beginning runner because it was flat, and I could run a circuitous pattern around the campus in 20 minutes. I gave each area a name: The Hidden Wood, The Quad, Parking, the Grand Entrance, and The Villas. The combination of aerobic activity, scenic beauty, and time to reflect made these runs addictive. I was recently divorced and trying to right myself after living sideways for so long. I listened to Dido and thought about life.

When I reached 30 minutes, I needed more space than campus could provide. I like to run a path only once instead of repeating a circuit or backtracking. I'd head out the back gate and into a large undeveloped area down below the campus. Dirt from construction sites was being dumped daily in the first section of it, so the landscape changed. At first, I skirted the piles but soon I was using them to increase my exertion, up one and down the next. A small creek started where the dirt dumping stopped, and I ran along it for a while, dodging willows, roots and rocks. The land rose in tiers on my right and as I became a stronger runner, I ran up and down those tiers. At the peak of my running career, I charged up all three of them and left the natural scenery for the city where I had to outrun stray dogs and dodge pot holes and bad drivers. That was an additional adrenaline rush.

"Take care of your body. It's the only place you have to live in."

—Jim Rohn

I was very aware of what running was doing to me physically first in the noise of my breathing, then the stretch of my thigh muscles and finally the throb of blood coursing through my veins. My head was also exercising, working out recent conflicts, then working through feelings about my divorce and 14-year marriage, and finally landing on the person I was becoming and would be. My heart benefited immensely from this. I forgave myself for falling in love with someone so wrong for me. I accepted praise for myself for taking care of my ex-husband for so long. I reconciled the person I was with the person I wanted to be. Running gave me a runner's body, and I enjoyed being fit.

I loved running in winter. It snowed a lot there and it stayed on the ground for long periods. My challenge became the corner near the entrance that always formed ice from the exhaust of the cars that stopped there. Could I round that corner without losing my footing and landing hard on my side? No. At least not very often, but I didn't change my route to avoid it. It was a talking point with other runners. I learned to respect people who do what I once thought were idiotic things like climbing Mt Everest. They must have started in the foothills. They must have started small. I imagine the health of their minds, bodies and hearts must tremendous. Learning how to be a runner taught me to be tolerant of behaviour I didn't understand.

Running in the spring meant running in the rain. Before becoming a runner, I thought people who ran in the rain were attention seekers, but I became one of them. As a runner, I was oblivious to other people. I was always so richly involved with the elements and my own body that people didn't exist. It must be true for most people who choose to exercise outside. They are not posing. They are engaged with the sublime. There's something liberating in running through the puddles because you're already so wet that it doesn't matter. Spring rains were sometimes warm and something cold, but they were always invigorating. Because I ran the same route daily, I could measure the growth of the buds. I was never a fast runner, so I could mark a plant on my path and study it daily. The path I was navigating internally was similar and noting the new growth of fruit trees, bulbs and even the grasses helped me reflect on my own growth. Now that I don't run, spring often surprises me.

I travelled in the summer, and ran on my travels. It's a great way to see a new city. I pushed myself up to 50 minutes when I was in Budapest, running to one bridge and crossing, then on to and around the island before crossing the bridge back and going past the Soviet monument and later St. Stephens. There were always other runners on this route, drawn, I suppose to the same things that drew me. I was a tourist, and they faces of the other runners showed them to be foreigners as well. Because runners always acknowledge one another, I felt like I was part of a global community. It's great to be in a club like that.

Autumn runs are yellow and my favorite. I learned to run in the spring, so by the time my first autumn as a runner arrived, I was a runner. I knew how to run, when to push, and when to slow down. It had become a great stabilizer in my life, and I will always associate autumn with this feeling: healthy mind, healthy heart, healthy body. Back on campus, I could choose the temperature. A cold run with hoody and gloves in the morning, or a hot, summer run in the afternoon. If I went as dusk approached, I started warm and then had to increase my pace as the cold crept back. I started the school year a different person, and that school year was my first as a runner.

"It is through the alignment of the body that I discovered the alignment of my mind, self, and intelligence."
—B.K.S. Iyengar

At the end of each run, I felt purged. Often a colleague would see me on my cool down and offer me a beer or a cup of coffee, depending on the person or the time of day. I was not a euphoric, diarrhoea-of-the-mouth-after-exercise kind of runner. Instead, I craved conversation with another person after so long in my own head and was a better listener than at other times in my day. I loved those post run chats, and because so many of us were in a similar place as me, less stressful jobs with more free time, those conversations could last for most of the morning or well into night.

Being outside is great for my mood. Getting aerobic exercise is great for my mood and my health. Being alone gives me time to reflect. Being outside, running alone brought me joy.

About Rita

Rita Roem lives in Colorado with her husband and two sons. She decided she wanted to be an English teacher when she was in the eighth grade and didn't look back until 20 years later when she had her own children to raise. She met her South African husband in Eastern Europe and together they enjoy the outdoor life that Colorado provides as well as traveling to cultural cities in America and Europe. She works within her community helping people who have autistic family and friends get connected to the services that they need.

Visit Rita at: https://turninginsideout.weebly.com

The Joy of Travel
by Maura Burgess

I was on an airplane the other day, and I struck up a conversation with a wonderful woman in the seat next to me. She mentioned that she had family all over the world. This particular trip, she was flying out to see one of her sons in Oklahoma. I thought it was amazing that her sons had lived all over the world and remarked that she must love to go and visit them. Her response shocked me. To her, traveling has no real allure, it is not a high point of her life, and she rarely engages in journeys outside her hometown. For someone like me, who literally hungers and thirsts to travel, whether it is across the ocean or across the street, this seemed like crazy talk! In fact, I informed her that I intended to walk on as much ground as possible and perhaps if I was very fortunate, meet a billion people. She smiled at me and wished me good luck on my goal.

So what is it, that makes me almost compulsive about seeking out new adventures and meeting new people? I think it all began on the eve of my fourth birthday. My father was in the military and we were being stationed in Germany. We flew from Miami, across the ocean, on a huge airplane. That was a very long time ago, because you could still smoke on flights. It was exciting, because it was my first flight. I vividly remember my father waking me up, and wishing me a happy birthday, as we flew over London. At that moment, I became very curious about all the cities that were below us.

My three years of life in Germany did not disappoint. I remember incredible festivals and awesome Christmas celebrations. I was especially impressed by the people. It was a delight to go into the local town, and have the shopkeepers set me on the counter, and bring me various treats. I also remember sitting on benches and locking arms with people and singing. This may or may not have had anything to do with Oktoberfest and beer. To me it was all a big, beautiful adventure. When we returned to the States, I made a promise to myself that I would see Europe again.

The moment was right, during the year of "celebrations". This was the year that I turned forty-five, my eldest son graduated high school, and my husband and I celebrated our twentieth wedding anniversary. Now, I believe in paying attention to what keeps appearing in your vision, spiritually and physically. Unexpectedly, the country of Croatia came up on our radar. Croatia, which used to be a part of

Yugoslavia, borders the Adriatic Sea and shares some common history with Italy. Through many conversations with world traveler friends, and after watching many Rick Steves' videos, we concocted a 16-day driving tour of Europe, with Croatia as the main focus. Somehow, through meditation and inquiries, the Croatian island of Vis, became a part of our itinerary. This little gem had vineyards, olive groves, and a complex history that involved ancient civilizations, secret military bunkers, and tunnels from its Yugoslavian past. We knew we could not pass up this adventure.

We arrived in the city of Split, Croatia and boarded a ferry for Vis. The boat ride was amazing. We went past many islands and enjoyed the views of the beautiful sea. I had rented an apartment from a woman named Mirsada, using an online service. She was waiting for us at the dock, holding up a sign, and smiling brightly. My husband and I, along with our two teenaged sons, followed along as she led us through steep and narrow streets, up the hillside to the apartment building. Even though we had packed pretty lightly, I felt like I was carrying boulders on my back! The 2-bedroom apartment was adorable. From there, we had a vantage point to watch vessels sail in and sail out. We could open the windows, and smell the Adriatic Sea, and hear all the wonderful sounds of the people, boats, and birds.

On our first evening, we wandered the streets, peeking at the menus of various cafes and restaurants. We finally settled on one restaurant that had a beautiful courtyard surrounded by lemon trees. It was amazing to sit in a place that had been around from the time of the Ancient Greeks. The owner brought out a big tray of fresh fish and we made a selection for our dinner. He had grown up on the island and was happy to tell us all about the history. He even introduced us to an enormous cat that ate all the extra scraps from the tables and the kitchen. When our food arrived, the waiter picked a lemon off of one of the trees nearby and squeezed it onto our seafood. We had a wonderful night drinking wine, eating delicious food and connecting with the locals.

On our second day, we went on a little boat for a cruise around the island. We were the only Americans. As we were sailing along, we were approached by a woman, named Nada. She was curious how we had ended up on the tiny island of Vis. She and her sister, Vlasta, were part of a Slovenian tour group and explained the history of Croatia and Slovenia. They had grown up when both countries were a part of Yugoslavia. It was amazing to learn so much from her about the background and culture of the region. Over the course of the day, we ate, we drank, we communed together, and a close friendship was formed. When we came back to the docks, we took photos as a group and we still exchange emails.

On our final evening, we strolled along the harbor and looked at all the sailboats, yachts, and dinghies. These sailors had come in from all over the world. On each boat, there was an abundance of singing, eating, drinking, and laughter. We were waved at by many people and invited to join in the fun, by a few. It was a perfect culmination of our time on Vis and affirmed why I love to travel. I had finally made it back to Europe and I was ready to go even further.

I realized that journeys are ultimately about finding the connection to other people and places. This brings me great joy and keeps me packing my suitcase. Every trip brings me a different perspective, no matter what the locale. From the food, to the lodging, to the new friendships, I get a window into how others live. This allows me to bring back new ideas and perspectives to my own life. I am so very grateful for my home base in Colorado. However, I will always be an explorer of sorts.

About Maura

Maura Burgess is a Spiritual/Life Comedian and Speaker that proudly displays her certificate from the Bovine Metropolis School of Improvisation and keeps her Accounting Degree hidden in a closet. She has served as a Spiritual Practitioner for the Centers for Spiritual Living and she facilitates The Mystical Traveling Sisters, a group of women who explore a variety of topics and spiritual modalities. Her calling is helping people to tap into their joyful, silly side and realize the power of showing up as "themselves. She is the creator the 'Sacred over Serious' experience, to encourage people to live boldly, joyfully and very irreverently (www.SacredOverSerious.com).

In Loving Memory of
Pedro Gonzalez, 1953-2016

Spiritual Joy from a Sundancers' Perspective:
An Interview with Pedro Gonzalez
by Joyce Graham

I was invited by Pedro to come to the annual Sundance in Arizona and to meet with him for this interview in the summer of 2015. The beauty of this drive from my home in Albuquerque, into northern New Mexico was breath taking. The hot sun of July beat down as I drove but the air was refreshing and I was excited. Kirsten and Pedro are newlyweds and I would be spending a few days with them at the Eagle Thunder/Sun Eagle sacred Sundance grounds. We were in the Red Valley of Arizona.

Upon arrival we had a sweat lodge and met many people. Wonderful meals and gatherings in the kitchen during my time there warmed my spiritual heart and set the gentle pace of this interview.

Joyce Graham: **Pedro can you tell me what brings you joy in your life?**
Pedro Gonzalez: Being able to help someone feel the oneness of connecting to our creator brings me great joy. When I am sharing a sweat lodge ceremony on the Sundance grounds, praying with my sacred pipe, dancing in the circle around the Sundance tree brings me joy. Having my new wife Kirsten experience this ceremony with me is a great blessing. It brings me much joy and happiness each year when we come here together.

JG: **Did you experience joy as a child?**
PZ: I was eight years old and my family was poor. My mother worked as a maid and my father as a gardener, pool cleaner and bar tender. We were happy even with little in the way of luxury. My first bike was a gift and it had no rubber tires to ride on. So, I rode only on the rims on the grass. This was pure joy.

JG: **Were their other "joys" as you were growing up?**
PZ: My sister took me at the age of fourteen to a spiritual temple in Mexico. One of the people there channeled a spirit. The spirit spoke to me and said "you are blessed with special energy". This person said I should use my gifts in the future to help people heal. This happened much later in my life because of course I was very young when this happened.

JG: **Have you had times in your life where you were not very joyful or happy?**

PZ: Yes, unfortunately I experienced sex, drugs and rock and roll. I was not committed in any way to my spiritual growth. When I turned thirty-five my life started changing. Gradually, I became more aware of my spiritual path. Practicing unconditional love and forgiveness became my focus. Now, for me the simple joys are the best. A smiling baby, and old couple holding hands, a beautiful sunset, lightning and rain, being with my partner, Kirsten. These are my true simple joys.

JG: **Are there times today that even with your spiritual practice do you feel the "blues"?**

PZ: Absolutely, I have down times. I feel when this happens to me I try to refocus my attention on the positive. I KNOW in my heart I am loved in my spiritual life and I speak this out loud. This is a very strong vibration and it changes us to say this. So, I practice this on a regular basis.

I believe we need to use "loving words" because this has a powerful vibration and effect on the people we are talking with. Using words and sound is an expression of great joy. Singing and drumming can create this healing as well.

JG: **Are there other ways you experience joy not yet mentioned?**

PZ: Yes, every year coming to Sundance is my biggest blessing. We start to prepare by making crowns, bracelets and anklets. While we do this preparation we are in communion with spirit. Internally, we are reviewing what moves us to commit to this strenuous ritual. The Sundancer believes he does this so that all his relations (plant kingdom, animal world, elements and spirit) may live. We share this knowledge with the new Sundancers that come every year.

People come from all over the US and different parts of the world each year to participate. Some dance others pray and observe. We all eat together, dance and pray together. There are rain storms, heat and simple joys that bond us together. This has been my life now for over eighteen years. Its pure happiness and joy to share in this sacred ceremony.

A Prayer

Aho, Tunkashila, Wankan Tanka. This is a Good Day to Die and a Good Day to Live. I give you Gratitude for allowing me to experience all the love that you send to all Creation.

Let me remember That We Are All One *so that I can be Loving and Understanding. That my awareness of your presence within me gives me the desire and ability to be of help to*

*others and myself. Let me be respectful towards
all my relations in the plant kingdom, animal
kingdom, mineral kingdom, all the elements
and the Spirit World so that my journey in this
beautiful river of life becomes an instrument of
your Devine Will.*

*Aho Mitakuye Oyasin
(We are all related)*

Mr. Bad hand facilitated his first experience on Hollow Horn Bear Sundance grounds in Rosebud, South Dakota. During his eighteen years living the Sundance experience he integrated the Lakota sacred ceremonies into his spiritual healing practice. With the help of his spirit friend Wakinya Wanbli (Eagle Thunder) and Archangels, Michael, Uriel, Jofiel, Zadkiel, Raphael, and Chamuel, he helped people to regain their mental, physical, emotional, and spiritual balance and health. www.sundancerhealer.com

Pedro Gonzalez lived and worked in Taos, New Mexico. He was born in 1953 to a lineage of Curanderas. In 1994 he moved to Taos where he was befriended by a well known Lakota Medicine Man, Mr. Howard Bad Hand. Prior to this meeting he received some spiritual gifts from his sister Lucy who is a conduit for the Tonantzin's energy.

Pedro left us in the Fall of 2016. He brought all who knew him the gift of unconditional love and his deeply healing spiritual work.

About Joyce

Joyce Graham is an author, educator, counselor, and Qi Gong Instructor. With over 30 years of experience in different countries all over the world, Joyce has a passion for helping people heal from the traumas of life, and realize their heart centered potential.

Joyce enjoys bringing other authors together to create works that are woven together to create beautiful "word tapestries." In her book, *The Path: Herbs, Homeopathy, Holistic Healing: A Resource Guide to Everyday Wellbeing,* Joyce created an anthology of knowledge-based writing from several leading practitioners , including herself, that is a guide to both the novice and expert.

In her first novel, *The Healer,* she creates endearing characters with which one becomes emotionally connected. It is a touching insight into the relationship between a mother with cancer and her daughter who is trying to help her by using both holistic natural medicine.

In her spare time, Joyce travels, enjoys walks in nature, cooking healthy meals, teaching Qi Gong and spending time with her friends and her significant other. She currently lives and has an office in Northern

Colorado. Cat Mandoo rules the house and often purrs on her lap while she writes.

Visit her website www.JoyceGraham.com
Or find her on her YouTube Channel

Contributing Authors

Maura Burgess is a Spiritual/Life Comedian and Speaker that proudly displays her certificate from the Bovine Metropolis School of Improvisation and keeps her Accounting Degree hidden in a closet. She has served as a Spiritual Practitioner for the Centers for Spiritual Living and she facilitates The Mystical Traveling Sisters, a group of women who explore a variety of topics and spiritual modalities. Her calling is helping people to tap into their joyful, silly side and realize the power of showing up as "themselves. She is the creator the 'Sacred over Serious' experience, to encourage people to live boldly, joyfully and very irreverently (www.SacredOverSerious.com).

John J. Candelaria describes himself as a narrative poet who enjoys writing poetry to capture the sound of language. In postic lines and free verse his poems have been published in *The Storyteller's Anthology*, Southwest Writers, The Oasis Journal 2012 and 2013, in the anthology, Poetry From The Other Side: an anthology, Albuquerque chapter, New Mexico State Poetry Society, and in the Southwest Sage newsletter of the SouthWest Writers.

Michael O. "Coop" Cooper is an internationally recognized executive coach, advisor, facilitator and trainer from San Francisco, California. He specializes in helping right-brain entrepreneurs recognize and monetize their brilliance to grow their companies. He founded Innovators + Influencers to help business leaders learn the skills, tools and strategies to thrive in a constantly changing environment. Even though he loves his work, he sneaks away for two weeks to the Burning Man festival in the Nevada Black Rock Desert every year to renew his spirit.

Visit Michael at: www.innovatorsandinfluencers.com

Pedro Gonzalez lived and worked in Taos, New Mexico. He was born in 1953 to a lineage of Curanderas. In 1994 he moved to Taos where he was befriended by a well known Lakota Medicine Man, Mr. Howard Bad Hand. Prior to this meeting he received some spiritual gifts from his sister Lucy who is a conduit for the Tonantzin's energy.

Pedro left us in the Fall of 2016. He brought all who knew him the gift of unconditional love and his deeply healing spiritual work.

Joyce Graham, MS, LPC is an author, presenter, Licensed Professional Counselor, and Qi Gong Instructor with over thirty years of experience. Her previous books include The Healer, a novel and The Path: Herbs, Homeopathy, Holistic Healing.

Visit her at www.JoyceGraham.com or on her YouTube Channel.

Andrea M. Hall is a certified Equine Gestalt Coach. She earned her certification through Melisa Pearce's program "Touched By A Horse". Through her own healing she and her horses are working with lawyers who may be at a crossroads in their life or just wanting to get off the hamster wheel of life. Couples who are struggling and wanting to determine what the next step in their relationship looks like. People who just want to heal old wounds and want to bring more peace and balance into their lives.

She has owned and operated a successful law firm specializing in sex offenses and domestic violence. Andrea is also a speaker and author of Sex and Justice. "Let the whisper of the horse echo the spirit of the soul."®

Visit Andrea at: www.witherswhisper.com

David Karchere is an author, speaker, poet, workshop leader and foremost thought leader on Primal Spirituality worldwide. David has created and led unique workshops for spiritual awakening and personal transformation for people around the globe. He has also developed The Creative Field Project, a global network of small groups that meet to further the work of Primal Spirituality. David has just finished writing his first book, *Becoming a Sun: Emotional and Spiritual Intelligence for a Happy, Fulfilling Life.*

David is a member of the Evolutionary Leaders group. His home is Sunrise Ranch in Loveland, Colorado, U.S.A., a teaching and demonstration site for Primal Spirituality.

Visit David at: www.davidkarchere.com

Rita Roem lives in Colorado with her husband and two sons. She decided she wanted to be an English teacher when she was in the eighth grade and didn't look back until 20 years later when she had her own children to raise. She met her South African husband in Eastern Europe and together they enjoy the outdoor life that Colorado provides as well as traveling to cultural cities in America and Europe. She works within her community helping people who have autistic family and friends get connected to the services that they need.

Visit Rita at: https://turninginsideout.weebly.com

Ruth Sharon, M.S. is a Licensed Professional Counselor, Registered Yoga Teacher and Sufi Healing Conductor. She and her husband Dr. Jim Sharon live in Centennial, CO and enjoy being with their family, friends and community.

Ruth and Jim have joyfully collaborated in writing the book *Secrets of a Soulful Marriage: Creating and Sustaining A Loving, Sacred Relationship,* SkyLight Paths Publishing,

2014. They offer personal counseling, as well as Coaching for Soulful Couples and Singles, retreats, seminars and a myriad of articles and interviews. They are voted "Best Relationship Coaches" in 2015 and 2016.

Visit Ruth at: www.energyforlife.us

Nick Zelinger spent 20 years as a touring musician, taught himself guitar, keyboards and bass guitar; opening for such music legends as The Vanilla Fudge, Strawberry Alarm Clock, and J.J. Cale. He recorded 3 albums with the eclectic folk rock band, Saxxon Woods. He continues to revel in the joys of making music, performing with the Denver-based rock band, Thin Ice (www.ThinIceBand.com).

Nick's has a successful career as a book designer, winning numerous national and international book awards (www.NZGraphics.com).

Nick is also the co-author, along with Tammy Brackett, of the award-winning book *Another Nightmare Gig from Hell, true stories from musicians across the country.* It is available on Amazon in softcover, eBook, and now in AudioBook format.

CPSIA information can be obtained
at www.ICGtesting.com
Printed in the USA
LVHW04235601018
592105LV00001B/187/P

9 780985 827922